# My Testimony

# And

# It's Benefits for You

## By Terry Board

© Burnett Publishing

2016

## Preface

I feel so blessed to be able to be writing this Preface. For two years I have been being treated by holistic means, diet and much prayer. I have listed many helps for you if you are a cancer patient or you know someone who is. Many good recipes are in the book as well. The greatest thing you can do for this disease is to have faith. One big piece of advice STAY OFF SUGAR! Cancer cells thrive on sugar. I hope this book serves as a blessing to all who read it.

Blessings,

Terry Board

## Endorsement:

*Terry Board has created a resource about cancer that it scriptural, spiritual and practical. Like the blind man who was healed by Jesus in John 9, Terry is giving God the praise and glory for her journey to healing.*

Robert Whitlow
Best-selling author of *A House Divided*

# Table of Contents

# MY TESTIMONY

## And its benefits for you

God has healed me of cancer. The one scripture that held me together was: Hebrews 11:6 *"Without **faith** it is impossible to please **God**, for you must believe that **God** is and that **God** is a rewarder of those who diligently seek Him!"* I give God ALL the glory for my healing!

My first priority was to please God and that meant believing that He is my God and that He would reward me because I was diligently seeking Him. Both my parents had cancer and they are both deceased now and many others in my family have had cancer and were treated with chemo and radiation. I have seen firsthand how it ravaged their bodies by killing everything inside, they had no immunity to fight off even a little cold. {My cousins wife had two sisters that had breast cancer at the same time and one took radiation and chemo, and the other chose holistic treatments. The one who chose chemo and radiation died and the other one is still living! That was about 12 years ago. Her life had given me hope.} So I decided that I would NOT have chemo and radiation, but would take the holistic way of healing. Most cancer can be reversed by diet alone but you have to be diligent about it. God has given us all things naturally to keep us well, but again we MUST be diligent at it, and of course I had many, many people praying for me. They stood with me and believed God to heal me through natural means and prayer.

*"**Faith** is the substance of things **hoped** for and the evidence of things NOT seen."* Take this scripture apart; what you are hoping for is the substance that faith creates. It takes that substance and turns it into evidence that has not even been seen yet! It may not look like anything has changed and symptoms may be screaming at you, but that doesn't mean God isn't working, or that He isn't there!

I want you to know that we can pray for people until the cows come home, but they have to join their faith with God and with yours. In Matthew the 9th chapter Jesus healed people over and over; *"Jesus turned and saw her. "Take heart, daughter," he said, "**your**

**faith has healed you**_." And the woman was healed at that moment."_ What did Jesus say healed her? He said her FAITH did it!

He healed some blind men. Scripture says; _"Then he touched their eyes and said, "According to **your faith** let it be done to you"; whose_ faith did Jesus say healed them? He said according to their faith! By the way what was their faith to be in? Faith in God!

Remember the man in the bible that said, "Lord I believe, help my unbelief?" One other thing I must tell you that God is a rewarder for those who diligently seek Him. He is a rewarder regardless of whether He heals you on this side of heaven or on the other side. After all the ultimate healing is to be with Him! God is good and His desire is to have you healed. Remember the scripture above? Some people get tired and they are ready to give up and go be with Jesus. It is according to their faith that it shall be done unto them.

So what is your faith? Are you believing, the symptoms? Are you believing, a death sentence from a doctor? Jesus paid a tremendous price for us to be healed, and scripture says "By His strips we ARE healed...even if it doesn't look like it at the moment.

You get what you say and what you believe! Proverbs 18:21 _"The tongue has the power of life and death, and those who love it will eat its fruit."_ What does this mean? It means you have what you speak and believe! Believe Gods word brothers and sisters!

I John 4:17 _"by this, love (What Love? His Love!) His love is perfected with us, that we may have confidence in the Day of Judgment; because as He is, so also are we in this world."_ The bible in the verses before the one I just quoted is talking about God's love. His love is perfected in us if we abide in Him and believe that He is God and we diligently seek Him. I know I sound like a broken record, but believe it … IT IS TRUE!

I Peter 1:3 _"Seeing that His divine power has granted to us everything pertaining to life and godliness, through the true knowledge of Him who called us by His own glory and excellence."_ Genesis 1:29 And God said, _"Behold, I have given you every plant yielding seed that is on the face of all the earth, and every tree with seed in its fruit."_
Here is why I say God has given us all things for our good. He has

given us <u>ALL</u> things pertaining to life...foods, flowers, herbs, seeds, nuts, vegetables, fruits, essential oils, and salts from beneath mountains. And before man got his hands on these things and changed their chemical make up with fertilizers, pesticides and other harmful chemicals, man used things in nature just as they are. Thousands of years ago there were no antibiotics. People cured themselves with plants from the earth. Even scripture tells us which animals we should eat and which ones we shouldn't.

Now I want to talk to you about the side of disease that makes you doubt. Believing is a full time job and if you let your guard down for one second the enemy will flood in. There will be times, you can hardly get through a day, but that is when you gather you arsenal of intercessory prayer partners that help believe with you and pray you through it. Even Moses who believed God to part the red sea had to have his arms held up. I have had to have my arms held up many times. Again going back to the scripture that held me, you know Hebrews 11:6 about diligently seeking God. Why do you suppose God said that... diligently seek Him? It is not a onetime fix and you are done, it is a process of seeking Him. Listen to these adjectives that describe diligent: painstaking, rigorous, careful, thorough. In order to do this you have to be responsible and reliable.

In "Life, Hope & Truth a publication Larry Murray writes: "*People with discipline have a goal, a vision of what is to be accomplished by their efforts. Keeping that vision in mind helps them stay focused and on task, even when the task at hand is laborious and tedious. Here is the strange truth: People without a vision or objective in life that they can diligently throw themselves into are inevitably unhappy. Larry Murray also reminds us of Jesus' promise in Revelation 2:10, "Be faithful until death, and I will give you a crown of life."*
Be patient, a seed takes time to grow, but once it does, it provides fruit for the season. I often speak of this. I used to tell my children about seeds, planting, watering and harvesting. Expect God to heal you! It may be a very long road. Even if the healing takes time, expect it.

In reference to all this I want to mention that it is all up to the person what they choose to do as far as their health is concerned. I am giving you what I did and others did it's up to you to do what you feel is right. I will not be responsible for someone using this information and then not following through and their situation getting worse. All I can assure you of is the word of God and all the scriptures you just read in this booklet. These words are truth and they are life. I do know that chemotherapy kills most of your good bacteria and all of the bad bacteria. I can with positive assurance tell you STAY AWAY from sugar if you have cancer! It feeds cancer and helps it grow.

As I just mentioned all scripture is truth and life. Proverbs 4:22 "My words are life to you, and health/medicine to all your flesh." Isaiah 57:19 "I will heal you." Read Psalm 103 it is full of good nuggets. I had to hold on for dear life to God's promises. As I said some days the pain was great and faith would start to falter. Brothers and sisters that scripture build your-self up in your most holy faith is so full of truth! I had to and then I'd call everyone I knew to pray. Not seeing anything happening for such a long time but knowing God was with me and that He would heal me according to my faith, kept me going. I could have been healed months before I had the test to show it. I just kept on believing that I was healed, and finally after my Hematologist/Oncologist said, "trust me on this one go get the mammogram, so I did. That doesn't mean I am totally in favor of mammograms. The ones now are much less evasive. They are three dimensional now also.

**Fasting** is another form of healing. Not only is it medically good for you but spiritually as well. Fasting causes you to detoxify and we all need detoxification. Isaiah the 58th chapter teaches you what a true fast is. Read it and ask God to examine your life...in other words shine a spot light on you to see if you are living according to this true fast. When you are diligently following this fast and God's promises in the 8th verse, that; your light shall break forth as the morning and your health shall spring forth speedily.

People with cancer need to have no stress in their lives. They need to have plenty of peace. Laugh a lot! The bible says "A merry heart is good like medicine." Get in at least (3) big belly laughs a day. Speak positive things. Make a notebook of all the positive scriptures you can find about your health, healing, finances and forgiveness. **Speak God's word** everyday about these things. **Forgiveness** plays an important role in your health as well. When you do not forgive you get rottenness in your bones. It will cause a whole plethora of diseases.

Bounce up and down or move your breast up and down often this helps your lymphatic system.

# Treatment Story

It all started with a mammogram back in 2014. They found a mass in my right breast. The radiologist did an ultrasound that looked suspicious and they wanted to do a biopsy to rule out breast cancer. I had been reading for a while about doctors saying do not get mammograms and do not let anyone cut on you in any way, not even a biopsy. If there was anything there, it could spread so I refused the biopsy. About two months went by before I did anything. All I had to go on was what I had seen and read about the terrible side effects of chemo and radiation. It was recommended that I have a thermography. I did have the Thermography and it revealed a clear mass in my left and right breast TH5 was found and this high rating showed at high risk that cancer is present. It was then recommended that I have an MRI of my breast to determine what stage. I couldn't afford an MRI and my insurance would not pay for it unless I had a biopsy. I began treatment with a holistic specialist. This consisted of acupuncture, totally getting off all medications, taking supplements, changing my diet radically, having sauna infrared treatments to help me detoxify, and magnetic treatments called PEMF (Pulsed Electromagnetic Field therapy). I had to get off DHEA which caused the overload of estrogen in my breast. I was told to never take it again. I had to begin a regimen of progesterone cream. Every night for a year I had to cover my breast before bed with castor oil and place a wool cloth over them with a heating pad for 20 minutes. Then spray an iodine solution on them and sleep with the iodine on.

I needed to get a confirmed diagnosis of the cancer so I paid over $100 to have a blood marker test CA 15-3 and 27-29 which confirmed a beginning stage 1 cancer. Normally these tests are done to those who have been diagnosed with metastatic cancer to see if treatments are responding correctly. http://emedicine.medscape.com/article/2087535-overview this is when we revved up my therapy. I was very diligent in staying with my diet and making the bone broth and drinking it twice a day. I truly believe that because we were on with my treatments so quickly that it did not allow the cancer to grow. I started feeling better than I had felt in years. Treatment continued for more than a year and a half I felt like it was gone but continued with the treatment. Then I went to see my Hematologist/Oncologist for my phlebotomy of my hemochromatosis. Hemochromatosis is when the body makes massive amounts of iron which can attack your liver, kidneys and heart. I already have paroxysmal ventricular tachycardia.  My heart rates jumps and speeds up rapidly even while sitting.  Recently my Hematologist/Oncologist did a very through breast exam while I was there before my phlebotomy and said he would really like for me to go get another mammogram because he didn't feel any signs of cancerous masses.  I really trust him so I did go back and have a mammogram.  They had me ready for an ultrasound after the mammogram and were planning on doing a biopsy.  I had many prayers going up that day and I prayed as well and while in the little waiting room I felt that I had been healed and they were not going to find anything.  The room I was in was **#3...Father, Son & Holy Spirit...The Trinity**!  The radiologist came in and said there is no need for an ultrasound there is <u>NO</u> sign of cancer.

## Some Practical Helps

Sip on lemon water throughout the day this also detoxifies you. Eat only farm feed free range chickens and eggs. Stay away from red meats. Make a bone soup with dried pea soup. Drink a cup of it in the morning and a cup at night. You can find the recipe in the recipe section. Eat nuts except peanuts. If you can't sleep at night eat an apple with almond butter which is a substitute for peanut butter. Stay away from wheat and all dairy. You can eat eggs if they are free range or cage free. Quinoa is a great grain that is acceptable to eat. Jasmine rice is a good rice to eat even though it is considered by some to be a starch. Eat fish from the sea especially any white fish. Cook it in the oven with some good spices. You can find out more in the appendices about spices. Mediterranean foods are great and so is most of the Paleo diet. NO SUGAR!!! Sweating helps get rid of toxins so don't be afraid to do some hard work and sweat or be in the sun with plenty of Sunscreen. Get a magnetic bracelet if you can't afford to go and have PEMF done at a holistic doctor's office. Drink plenty of green tea. Drink (2) cups of dandelion tea, it has been reported that some people with stage 4 cancer have drank this tea for a period of (3) to (4) months and have been totally been cured from cancer. Get it from a health food store buy organic. Some people dig it up out of their yards. I didn't because it can have chemicals from lawn care on it.

Simple things like taking a tablespoon of cinnamon and honey will relieve pain and inflammation. It takes not more than a half teaspoon of cinnamon powder every day to keep cancer risk away. A natural food preservative, cinnamon is a source of iron and calcium. Useful in reducing tumor growth, it blocks the formation of new vessels in the human body. There is much more in the appendices that list information about diet, spices, herbs and supplements that not only are good for you but, actually heal you.

The ability of cinnamon extracts to suppress the in vitro growth of **H. pylori**, a recognized risk factor for gastric cancer, gastric mucosa-associated lymphoid tissue lymphoma, and pancreatic cancer, has stirred considerable interest in the potential use of this spice to suppress human cancers (Farinha and Gascoyne 2005; Eslick 2006).

Keep your body at a PH alkaline level 7.4 to 8.0. Get Hydrion Test papers from Walmart and check your PH every other day.

# Oil Pulling

Oil Pulling is an ancient cleansing and detoxifying technique.

First thing in the morning on an empty stomach, before brushing your teeth and before drinking any liquids (including water) or eating, pour **one tablespoon of coconut oil or sesame seed oil (or whatever oil you have chosen, organic preferred)** into your mouth.
I prefer coconut oil.

Swish the oil around in your mouth **without swallowing** it.  Move it around in your mouth and through your teeth, as if it was mouthwash. (**Don't tilt your head back to gargle**.)  You'll find that the oil will start to get watery as your saliva mixes with it.  Keep swishing.

If your jaw muscles get sore while swishing, you're putting too much into it.  Relax your jaw muscles and use your tongue to help move the liquid around the inside of your mouth.  When you do this correctly, you'll feel very comfortable.

There is no right way or wrong way to swish and pull oil.  Don't focus on doing it right.  Do it with very natural movement.  Do this gently, in a relaxed way **for about 10 minutes**.

**VERY IMPORTANT**:  Spit the oil out in the trash (do not spit in sink/drain/toilet...IT WILL clog the pipes), then rinse your mouth with water.

You can repeat at noon on empty stomach.

*Helpful Information:*

# Breast Cancer Index Test

Sign in to receive recommendations (Learn more
Once you create an account at Breastcancer.org, you can
enter information about your breast cancer diagnosis (e.g.
breast cancer stage), plan your treatments, and track your
progress through treatments. Based on your unique
information, Breastcancer.org can recommend articles that
are highly relevant to your situation.)

The Breast Cancer Index test, made by bioTheranostics,
analyzes the activity of seven genes to help predict the risk of
node-negative, hormone-receptor-positive breast cancer
coming back 5 to 10 years after diagnosis. The test can help
women and their doctors decide if extending hormonal
therapy 5 more years (for a total of 10 years of hormonal
therapy) would be beneficial.  The Breast Cancer Index
reports two scores: how likely the cancer is to recur 5 to 10
years after diagnosis and how likely a woman is to benefit
from taking hormonal therapy for a total of 10 years.

Research suggests the Breast Cancer Index test may
eventually be widely used to help make treatment decisions
based on the cancer's risk of coming back in a part of the
body away from the breast (distant metastasis) within 10
years after diagnosis.

Right now, the Breast Cancer Index test is not approved by
the U.S. Food and Drug Administration.

# What are genomic tests?

Genomic tests analyze a sample of a cancer tumor to see how
active certain genes are. The activity level of these genes
affects the behavior of the cancer, including how likely it is to

grow and spread. Genomic tests are used to help make make make decisions about whether more treatments after surgery would be beneficial.

While their names sound similar, genomic testing and genetic testing are very different.

Genetic testing is done on a sample of your blood, saliva, or other tissue and can tell if you have an abnormal change (also called a mutation) in a gene that is linked to a higher risk of breast cancer. See the Genetic Testing pages for more information.

## Who's eligible for the Breast Cancer Index test?

You may be eligible for the Breast Cancer Index test if:

- you were diagnosed with early-stage (stage I-III) breast cancer
- the cancer was hormone-receptor-positive and HER2-negative
- there was no cancer in your lymph nodes (lymph node-negative disease)
- you've been taking hormonal therapy for 4 to 5 years and want to know if taking hormonal therapy for more time will be beneficial

Research has shown that extending hormonal therapy for 5 more years — for a total of 10 years of hormonal therapy — can offer benefits for some women diagnosed with early-stage, hormone-receptor-positive, HER2-negative disease.

The Breast Cancer Index test is performed on preserved tissue that was removed during the original biopsy or surgery.

Because many women have troubling side effects, including hot flashes and joint pain, from hormonal therapy, they want to know if extending the time they take hormonal therapy is worth tolerating the side effects.

## How does the Breast Cancer Index test work?

The Breast Cancer Index genomic test analyzes the activity of seven genes that can influence how likely the cancer is to come back 5 to 10 years after diagnosis, as well as how likely a woman is to benefit from 5 additional years of hormonal therapy.

The Breast Cancer Index test results have two scores:

- The BCI Prognostic score estimates how likely the cancer is to come back 5 to 10 years after diagnosis (late recurrence). Scores range from 0 to 10. Cancers with scores of 0 to 5 are classified as having low risk of late recurrence. Cancers with scores of 5.1 to 10 are classified as having a high risk of late recurrence.
- The BCI Predictive score estimates how likely a woman is to benefit from taking hormonal therapy for 5 more years for a total of 10 years. The results are reported as either low likelihood of benefit or high likelihood of benefit.

## Insurance coverage and financial assistance

The Medicare program and several other major insurance companies have agreed to cover the Breast Cancer Index test. BioTheranostics, the company that makes the Breast Cancer Index test, has a Patient Advocates Team to help you with verifying insurance coverage and obtaining reimbursement. The company also has a patient assistance program that helps pay for testing. To contact the Patient Advocates Team, call 858-587-5886, Monday through Friday, 7 a.m.-4 p.m. Pacific Time.

# Other genomic tests

There are other genomics tests used to analyze breast cancer tumors. To learn more, click on the links below.

- The EndoPredict test is used to predict the risk of distant recurrence of early-stage, hormone-receptor-positive, HER2-negative breast cancer that is either node-negative or has up to three positive lymph nodes.
- The MammaPrint test is used to predict the risk of recurrence within 10 years after diagnosis of stage I or stage II breast cancer that is hormone-receptor-positive or hormone-receptor-negative.
- The Mammostrat test is used to predict the risk of recurrence of early-stage, hormone-receptor-positive breast cancer.
- The Oncotype DX test is used to predict the risk of recurrence of early-stage, hormone-receptor-positive breast cancer, as well as how likely it is that a woman diagnosed with this type of cancer will benefit from chemotherapy after surgery. The Oncotype DX DCIS test is used to predict the risk of recurrence of DCIS and/or the risk of a new invasive cancer developing in the same breast, as well as how likely it is that a woman diagnosed with DCIS will benefit from radiation after surgery.
- The Prosigna Breast Cancer Prognostic Gene Signature Assay (formerly called the PAM50 test) is used to predict the risk of distant recurrence for postmenopausal women within 10 years of diagnosis of early-stage, hormone-receptor positive disease with up to three positive lymph nodes after 5 years of hormonal therapy.

Breast MRI (Magnetic Resonance Imaging)

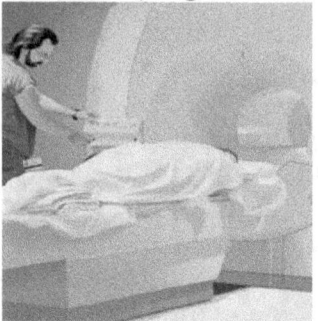

MRI, or magnetic resonance imaging, is a technology that uses magnets and radio waves to produce detailed cross-sectional images of the inside of the body. MRI does not use X-rays, so it does not involve any radiation exposure. Breast MRI has a number of different uses for breast cancer, including:

- screening high-risk women (women known to be at higher than average risk for breast cancer, either because of a strong family history or a gene abnormality)
- gathering more information about an area of suspicion found on a mammogram or ultrasound
- monitoring for recurrence after treatment

**SPICES**

Turmeric and cumin are known for being great pain relievers and also for reducing inflammation. You can also get that from a health food store.

## Natural Pain Relief: Popular Herbal Options
Here are some common herbal remedies used for natural pain relief:

- By: Juhie Bhatia | Medically reviewed by Kevin O. Hwang, MD, MPH
- Online Magazine Everyday Health

- **Capsaicin.** Derived from hot chile peppers, topical capsaicin may be useful for some people in relieving pain. "Capsaicin works by depleting substance P, a compound that conveys the pain sensation from the peripheral to the central nervous system. It takes a couple of days for this to occur," says David Kiefer, MD, assistant clinical professor of medicine at the Arizona Center for Integrative Medicine.

- **Ginger.** Though more studies are needed, says Dr. Kiefer, ginger extract may help with joint and muscle pain because it contains phytochemicals, which help stop inflammation. Few side effects have been linked to ginger when taken in small doses.

- **Feverfew.** Feverfew has been used for centuries to treat headaches, stomachaches, and toothaches. Nowadays it's also used for migraines and rheumatoid arthritis. More studies are required to confirm whether feverfew is actually effective, but the herb may be worth trying since it hasn't been associated with serious side effects. Mild side effects include canker sores and irritation of the tongue and lips. Pregnant women should avoid this remedy.

- **Turmeric.** This spice has been used to relieve arthritis pain and heartburn, and to reduce inflammation. It's unclear how turmeric works against pain or inflammation, but its activity may be due to a chemical called curcumin, which has anti-inflammatory properties. Turmeric is usually safe to use, but high doses or long-term use may cause indigestion. Also, people with gallbladder disease should avoid using turmeric.

- **Devil's Claw.** There is some scientific evidence that this South African herb may be effective in managing arthritis and lower back pain, but more research is needed. Side effects are very rare if taken at a therapeutic dose for the short term, but it's not advised for pregnant women and those with gallstones or stomach or intestinal ulcers.

## Natural Pain Relief: Proceed With Caution

There are many other herbal remedies for natural pain relief, such as boswellia and willow bark. The American Pain Foundation also lists these herbs for pain management:

- **Ginseng** for fibromyalgia
- **Kava Kava** for tension headaches and neuropathic pain
- **St. John's Wort** for sciatica, arthritis, and neuropathic pain
- **Valerian root** for spasms and muscle cramps

Since herbal therapies for pain management have yet to be thoroughly studied, be careful when embarking on this treatment path. Regardless of the herb you try, remember that they're not benign. Research into their safety and efficacy is still limited, and the government doesn't regulate herbal products for quality. The best course is to talk to a health-care professional before testing out a herbal remedy.

Last Updated: 2/10/2016

http://naturalsociety.com/16-natures-best-natural-pain-killers/

http://www.prevention.com/mind-body/natural-remedies/pain-remedies-natural-cures-pain

http://www.organiclifestylemagazine.com/foods-vitamins-and-herbs-that-kill-cancer

https://www.collective-evolution.com/2014/03/26/this-little-known-chinese-herb-kills-12000-cancer-cells-for-every-healthy-cell/

Your holistic specialist will also have herbs and a list of what you should eat.

If you are in Charlotte here are a few references to Holistic practice:

Trinity Chiropractic & Natural Medicine off of Independence Blvd just after crossing over I-485 on the right.  Dr. Hojoon Song, DC,MS, MS  704-684-0093  He is a naturopathic specialist.

http://www.charlottenaturalhealing.com/about/meet-dr-jeremy/

http://lifestyle-clinic.com/services/naturopathic-medicine-charlotte/    I do not know this clinic myself, but heard that it was a good source for many naturopathic illnesses.

# APPENDEX 2

## SPICES AND FOODS

There are numerous spices that control cancer; below are a few links for you to check out.

http://www.realnews24.com/18-spices-scientifically-proven-to-prevent-and-treat-cancer/

http://www.earthespice.com.au/blog/this-is-what-happens-to-your-body-if-you-eat-1-teaspoon-of-turmeric-every-day/

### Ginger:

Another weapon in your kitchen's cancer prevention arsenal, fresh ginger contains gingerol while dried ginger forms zingerone. "Gingerol and zingerone are thought to have antioxidant and anti-inflammatory properties, and therefore may be protective against cancer," explains Bethany Smith, RD, a nutritionist at Georgia Cancer Specialists in Atlanta. Store ginger in the freezer and grate a bit into lentils or rice when cooking. Steeping a few thin slices in hot water for 10 to 15 minutes can create a calming tea that may help with nausea and also decrease cancer risk.
Another weapon in your kitchen's cancer prevention arsenal, fresh ginger contains gingerol while dried ginger forms zingerone. "Gingerol and zingerone are thought to have antioxidant and anti-inflammatory properties, and therefore may be protective against cancer," explains *Bethany Smith, RD, a nutritionist at Georgia Cancer Specialists in Atlanta.* Store ginger in the freezer and grate a bit into lentils or rice when cooking. Steeping a few thin slices in hot water for 10 to 15 minutes can create a calming tea that may help with nausea and also decrease cancer risk.

### Garlic

Along with onions, shallots, scallions, and leeks, garlic is an allium vegetable that may help prevent cancer, especially of the stomach.  Allium vegetables contain oregano-sulfur compounds, the chemical that causes eye-tearing when they're chopped. Oregano-sulfur has immune-strengthening, Anti-carcinogenic qualities. Garlic is a versatile cooking essential. It can be sautéed in a tablespoon of olive oil and served with whole grain bread, or baked in the oven and then mashed into a spread. It's delicious added to vegetables and meats dishes.

## Turmeric

The spice turmeric contains curcumin, which gives curry powder its yellow color. "Curcumin is one of the most powerful anti-inflammatories identified to this day," says *Amanda Bontempo, RD, CDN, an ambulatory oncology dietitian at Montefiore Medical Center in the Bronx, N.Y.*

Cancer tumors have a network of blood vessels that feed them, explains Bontempo, and curcumin can work against these blood vessels and essentially choke the cancer cells to death. Mixing tumeric with black pepper and olive oil can activate curcumin's power. With its mild and pleasant flavor, Turmeric can be used as a dry rub on chicken or even vegetables. A teaspoon or two can also be added to soups, sauces, or stews — a tasty way to practice cancer prevention.

http://www.ncbi.nlm.nih.gov/books/NBK92774/

http://www.naturallivingideas.com/19-herbs-spices-that-fight-cancer/

Continued is a list of Recipes.

# RECIPES

**Some recipes I got from friends and I do not know where they got them from**

# Carrot Ginger Soup Recipe

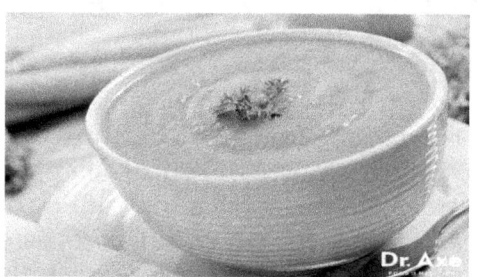

This carrot ginger soup is delicious! It's full of **vitamin A**, nutrients and flavor that is sure to please all! Add it to a meal or enjoy it by itself! Those soup can be served both hot and chilled!

**Total Time:** 60 minutes   **Serves:** 8

## INGREDIENTS:

- 2 pounds carrots, chopped
- 2 onions, peeled and chopped
- 5-7 cups **chicken broth**
- 3 tbsp fresh ginger, grated
- 3 garlic cloves, chopped
- 1 cup kefir
- **Sea Salt, Black Pepper** and **Onion Powder** to taste
- 2-3 tbsp **ghee**

## DIRECTIONS:

1. Place carrots, bone broth, ginger, and garlic in a pot and bring to a boil. Reduce heat and simmer until carrots are soft when pierced.

2. Saute onions in a separate pan with ghee over medium high heat until caramelized.

3. Add both the broth mixture and the onions to a blender and blend until a smooth consistency is reached. (You may have to do this in more than 1 batch)

4. Transfer smooth mixture back into large pot and add kefir and seasonings. Mix until well incorporated.

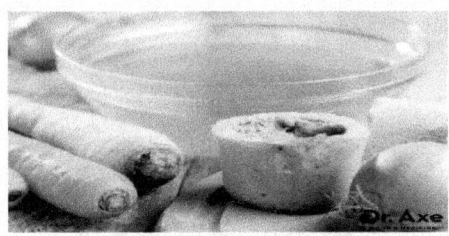

# Beef Bone Broth Recipe

**Total Time:** 48 hours  **Serves:** Varies

## INGREDIENTS:

- Beef bones with marrow
- water to cover bones
- 3 tbsp **apple cider vinegar**
- 2 Bay Leaves
- Sea Salt and Ground Black Pepper
- vegetables of choice

## DIRECTIONS:

1. Place all ingredients in crockpot. Add in water until bones are covered.

2. Turn setting to high and let simmer for 48 hours

# BONE BROTH
## The one I used mostly
### Broth Ingredients

6 Shitake mushrooms

1 Reishi mushroom (Lingzhi mushroom) mushroom

6 pieces Astragalus root

4 carrots

1 bunch parsley

1 lb. Ox tail

1 oz. Maitake

1 piece Kombu

1 large yellow onions

### Consider adding one or all of the following:

Spinach (558 mg potassium/100 grams)     Beet greens (762 mg potassium/100 grams)

Kale (447 ms potassium/100 grams)

In 1 gallon **DISTILLED** water, in order to get the full benefit of the high potassium in the broth); add all ingredients; bring to a boil; then let simmer for **10 to 24** hours; the strain.

{I just used one of the mushrooms, whichever one I could find. Then just remove the mushrooms and the ox tail.  Next I had 10 mason jars and filled them up and put them in the refrigerator I would take one out a day and drink half in the morning and half in the evening,}

***You can drink a whole jar twice a day if you'd like.

*** You can add minced garlic to the broth also.

The broth also needs either salt (sea salt) or miso (It is fabulous with a tablespoon of miso.)

Use the broth also to cook with, as a base for chicken soup or just use it as a fasting meal.  This broth will help boost up your immune system.  Try to drink 2-5 cups a day.

You can find of some of the ingredients at most Asian Markets.

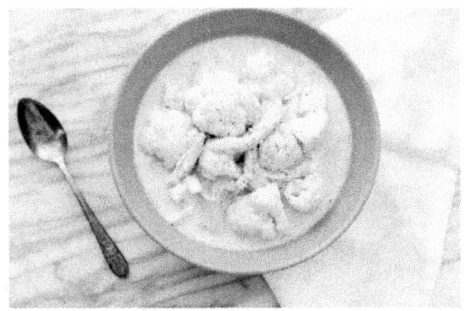

# Curried Cauliflower Soup

**Total Time:** 40 minutes/Serves: 6–8

INGREDIENTS:

- 1 tablespoon grass-fed butter or coconut oil
- 1 head cauliflower, cut into medium pieces
- 1 leek, chopped, white and green parts separated
- 2 medium kohlrabi, peeled and diced
- 4 cups low-sodium chicken broth
- 1/2 teaspoon salt
- one 2-inch knob of turmeric, peeled, washed and grated
- one 2-inch knob of ginger, peeled, washed and grated
- 2 tablespoons curry powder of your choice: yellow, Maharajah, Ras el Hanout, etc
- 1–2 teaspoons cayenne pepper (optional)
- juice and zest of 1 lemon, divided
- 5 cloves garlic, minced or pressed
- meat from 1 rotisserie chicken, pulled
- two 13.5-ounce cans coconut milk
- 1 tablespoon coconut sugar (optional)

## DIRECTIONS:

1. In a large pot or dutch oven, heat the butter or oil over medium heat until the butter is melted or the oil is shimmering.

2. Add the cauliflower, white parts of the leek and the kohlrabi. Saute for 5–8 minutes, stirring often.

3. Increase heat to medium-high. Add the chicken broth, salt, turmeric, ginger, curry powder and optional cayenne pepper. Cover and bring soup to a low boil.

4. Once the soup is boiling, stir in the lemon juice, green parts of the leek, garlic, chicken, coconut milk and optional coconut sugar. Decrease the heat to low and simmer for 10 minutes.

5. Taste the soup and add more salt if needed. Simmer for 10 minutes more. Remove the pot from heat and stir in the lemon zest. Allow soup to rest for 5 minutes before serving. Soup flavor will continue to improve over the next few days.

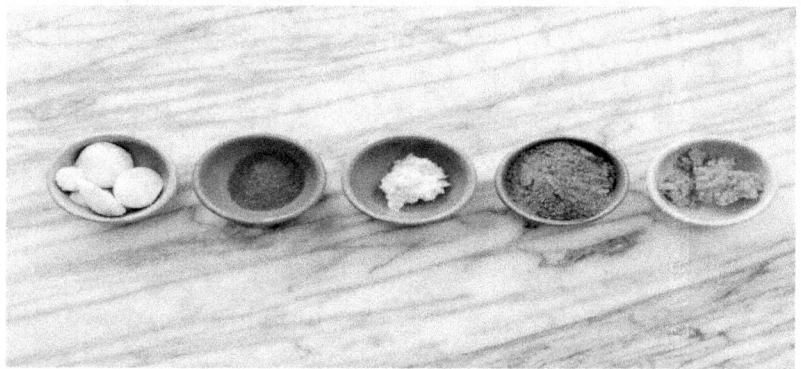

Does seeing "curried" in a recipe title intimidate you? Indian recipes can have a reputation for being complicated or difficult, but most of the time I think we're just thrown off by all those spices we're not accustomed to using. **Curry** dishes can actually be super simple and quick to make, with tons of flavor and health benefits.

Take this Curried Cauliflower Soup, for example. What's less intimidating than a soup? Throw everything together, let it simmer, and then sit back and be wowed by your creation. It all centers around **cauliflower**, one of the world's healthiest vegetables that chockfull of both phytochemicals and anti-inflammatories.

My Curried Cauliflower Soup is great because you can use leftover chicken or meat from a prepared rotisserie chicken — that's one big step cut out right there! You can even make this soup meat-free: All the veggies and creamy coconut milk will fill you up and leave you satisfied. **Benefit-rich turmeric**, ginger and curry also not only help you feel full, but they aid in digestion, improve circulation, and reduce cholesterol and inflammation among many other benefits.

Combine those super spices with garlic, **cayenne pepper** and cauliflower, and this soup is your immune system's new best friend. Now let's get to simmering...

First you'll want to prep all of your veggies: cauliflower, leek and kohlrabi. Kohl-what? Kohrabi, also called "turnip cabbage," is that funky-looking vegetable that you see come into season starting in October. Its texture and flavor are similar to a broccoli stem but sweeter. Cooking it brings out even more of its natural sweetness, but what's really sweet are all its nutrients: vitamin C, potassium, fiber, magnesium and iron. Be sure to remove the tough outer layer before dicing it up.

Leeks are our stand-in for onions in this soup. You'll love the sweet flavor they impart, too. Just make sure you clean leeks well before using them.

Then start with a large soup pot over medium heat. Add your butter or oil and get it nice and hot. Throw in the cauliflower, the white parts of the leek and the kohlrabi. Stir them around and saute for 5 to 8 minutes. You want to begin to bring out the veggies' flavors and get a little color on them. **By Dr. Josh Axe**

After the veggies have sautéed for a bit, turn the heat up to medium-high and add in the chicken broth, salt and spices. Now your kitchen is going to start smelling amazing. Cover the soup and bring it to a boil. This would be a great time to pull apart your chicken if needed.

Once the soup is boiling, add in the juice of 1 lemon, the green parts of the leek, all that delicious minced garlic, pulled chicken and 2 cans of full-fat **coconut milk**. If you'd like to balance the spices with a bit of sweetness, add in 1 tablespoon of coconut sugar here. Decrease the heat to low and allow the soup to simmer, uncovered, for 10 minutes. You'll see it begin to reduce and thicken.
Taste the soup at this point and add salt if you'd like. Then simmer it for 10 minutes more.

To finish the soup, remove the pot from the heat and stir in the lemon zest. This is going to give you a punch of fresh flavor right at the end. Cover the soup and let it rest for 5 minutes. Then ladle it up and enjoy your Curried Cauliflower Soup. You made a curry dish! That wasn't difficult at all, was it?

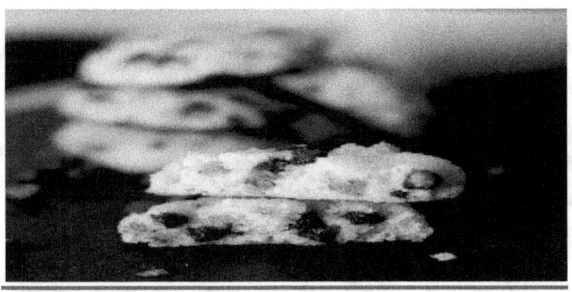

# Coconut Flour Chocolate Chip Cookies
## (Grain-free)
makes 12 cookies

**Adapted from** *this recipe*

## Ingredients:

1/3 cup coconut flour
1/4 cup coconut oil, melted
1/4 cup pure maple syrup
1 teaspoon vanilla extract
1/4 teaspoon salt
2 whole eggs
1/3 cup dark chocolate chips

## Directions: below

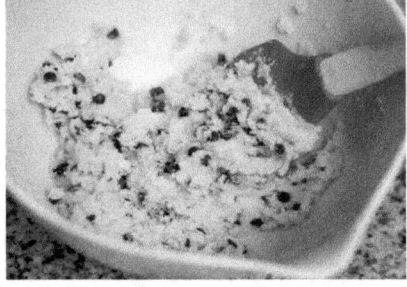

Use a heaping tablespoon to drop the cookie dough onto the lined baking sheet, and use your hands to flatten the cookies. Keep in mind these cookies will NOT spread on their own, so you'll want to shape them how you'd like them to turn out.

Bake at 350F for 12-14 minutes, until the edges are golden brown. Allow to cool on the pan for 10 minutes, then transfer to a wire rack to cool completely.

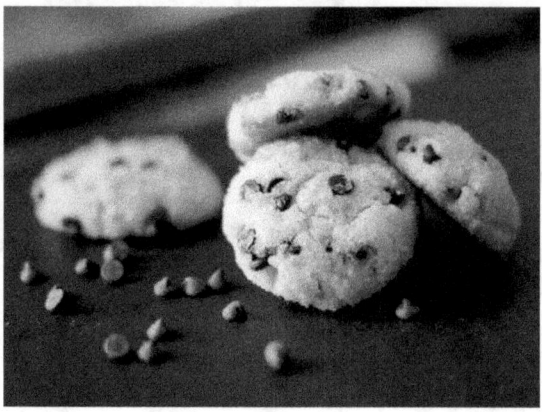

*Note: These cookies can be stored on the counter for a few days, but I found that they get even softer after a few days at room temperature, so they are best stored in the fridge for the longest shelf life.

### Ingredients

- ⅓ cup coconut flour
- ¼ cup coconut oil, melted
- ¼ cup pure maple syrup
- 1 teaspoon vanilla extract
- ¼ teaspoon salt
- 2 whole eggs
- ⅓ cup dark chocolate chips

### Instructions

1. Preheat your oven to 350F and line a baking sheet with a Silpat or parchment paper.
2. In a medium bowl, whisk together the coconut flour, coconut oil, maple syrup, vanilla, salt and eggs until a uniform batter is created. The batter will start off a bit runny, but will thicken as the coconut flour starts to absorb the moisture. Add in the chocolate chips, and stir to distribute them evenly. (I used Enjoy Life allergen-free mini chocolate chips in this particular batch.)
3. Use a heaping tablespoon to drop the cookie dough onto the lined baking sheet, and use your hands to flatten the cookies. Keep in mind these cookies will NOT spread on their own, so you'll want to shape them how you'd like them to turn out.

4.  Bake at 350F for 12-14 minutes, until the edges are golden brown. Allow to cool on the pan for 10 minutes, and then transfer to a wire rack to cool completely.

As I mentioned above, there is no substitute for coconut flour. If you want to use a different type of flour, I'd recommend trying my chocolate chip cookie recipes using <u>almond flour</u> or <u>buckwheat flour</u>, instead.

- I don't recommend trying to use flax eggs as a substitute for the whole eggs in this recipe. I tried it myself, and the resulting cookies were mushy and wouldn't come off the pan.
- Feel free to use honey, instead of maple syrup, if you like; keeping in mind that honey is sweeter, so you'll need to use less of it.

Enjoy! **By Dr. Josh Axe**

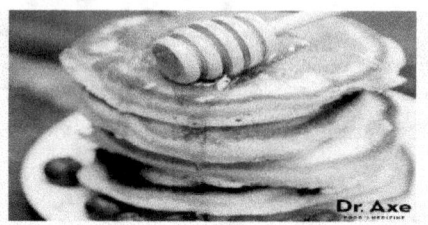

# Flour-less Pancakes Recipe

**Total Time:** 15 minutes   **Serves:** 1

INGREDIENTS:

- 2 ripe bananas, mashed
- 3 eggs
- 1 tsp **cinnamon**
- 1 tsp **vanilla extract**
- **sea salt** to taste
- Ghee

DIRECTIONS:

1. Combine all ingredients in a bowl
2. Pour batter into a pan with melted ghee over medium heat. Cook until small bubbles form and then flip.

Recipe by Dr. Axe

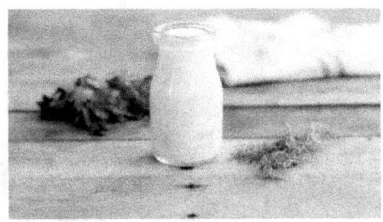

# Homemade Ranch Dressing

**Total Time:** 5 minutes/**Serves:** 4–6

- 2 cloves garlic, pressed or minced
- 1/4 teaspoon sea salt or smoked salt
- 1 cup Vegenaise
- 1/4 cup coconut cream
- 1/4 cup fresh parsley
- 2 tablespoons fresh dill
- 2 tablespoons fresh chives
- 1 teaspoon Worcestershire sauce
- 1/2 teaspoon black pepper
- 1 teaspoon coconut vinegar
- 1/2 teaspoon paprika
- 1/2 teaspoon cayenne

DIRECTIONS:

1. In a small bowl, combine all ingredients and mix well. Store in a sealed container in the refrigerator for up to 7 days.

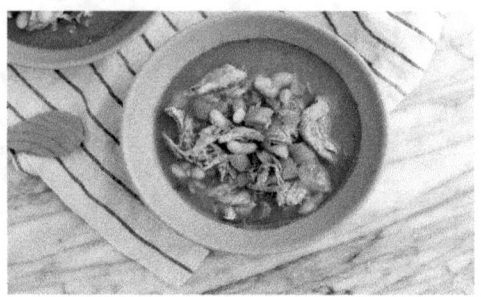

# White Chicken Chili

**Total Time:** 1 hour 15 minutes/**Serves:** 6–8

- 3 boneless skinless chicken breasts, at room temperature
- 4 tablespoons melted coconut oil, divided
- 2 small yellow onions, diced
- 1/4 red onion, diced
- 1 red bell pepper, diced
- 1 jalapeno pepper, seeded and diced
- 2 cloves garlic, peeled and diced
- 2 teaspoons cumin
- 2 teaspoons chili powder
- 1 teaspoon smoked paprika
- 2 cups chicken broth
- one 28-ounce can whole, peeled, fire-roasted tomatoes with juice
- one 14-ounce can cannellini beans, drained and rinsed
- salt and pepper to taste

DIRECTIONS:

1. Heat the oven to 425 F. Line a baking sheet with parchment paper.

2. Rub the chicken breasts with 2 tablespoons of the coconut oil and season with salt and pepper. Place on the lined baking sheet and bake for 25 minutes. While the chicken is baking, prepare the soup.

3. In a large soup pot over medium-high heat, heat the remaining 2 tablespoons of coconut oil until it shimmers. Add the onions, bell pepper, jalapeno, garlic, cumin, chili powder and paprika. Cook for 8 minutes, stirring frequently, until the onions are soft.

4. Stir in the chicken stock and fire-roasted tomatoes. Increase the heat to high and bring the mixture to a boil. Boil for 2 minutes. Reduce the heat to low, cover and simmer for 35 minutes.

5. Remove the chicken from the oven and allow it to cool slightly. Using two forks, pull apart   the chicken into bite-size pieces.

6. With a wooden spoon, break apart the tomatoes in the chili. Stir in the beans and the chicken. Cover and simmer for 20 more minutes.

7. Allow the soup to rest for 10 minutes. Add salt and pepper to taste. Serve topped with a lime wedge, cilantro or both.

Chili is one of those foods you can't go wrong with — there are so many varieties to choose from! There's **bison chili, buffalo chili** and even **turkey chili with adzuki beans**. But I'll let you in on a secret: this White Chicken Chili recipe is my new favorite for the winter. It puts a new spin on the typical chili recipe by using chicken breasts and cannellini beans for a whole lot of protein and flavor. Best of all, this white chicken chili recipe comes together in under 90 minutes. No more waiting all day to get a bowl of chili on the table.  Ready to try this new take on an old favorite?

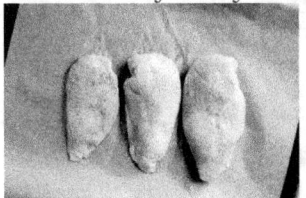

Start by heating the oven to 425 F and lining a baking sheet with parchment paper. While the oven heats up, drizzle the chicken breasts with 2 tablespoons of coconut oil and season with salt and pepper to taste. Place them on the baking sheet and slide that chicken into the oven. As it bakes for the next 25 minutes, we're going to get that soup started.

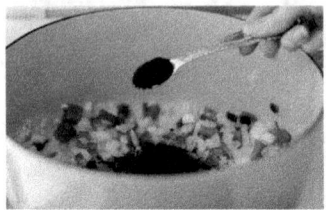

Grab a large soup pot and, over medium-high heat, heat the other 2 tablespoons of coconut oil until it's nice and shimmery. Then add in the nutrition-rich onions, bell pepper, jalapeno, garlic, cumin, chili powder and paprika. I love how colorful this white chicken chili is, as it's an indication of how good it is for your plus makes it more interesting to cook and eat.

Cook that up for 8 minutes, steadily stirring the ingredients, until the onions are nice and soft.

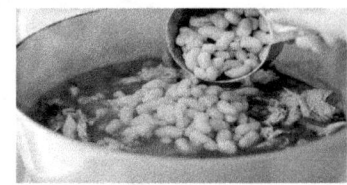

Once the onions have softened, it's time to add the rest of the good stuff. Stir in the chicken stock and fire-roasted tomatoes. Crank the heat up and bring the pot to a boil for 2 minutes. Then lower the heat to low, cover and let all the flavors simmer for 35 minutes.

The chicken should be cooked by now. Remove it from the oven and let it cool until it won't burn your fingers. Then, using two forks (or your fingers if you're up for it!), shred the chicken into bite-sized pieces.

Next, grab a wooden spoon and break apart the tomatoes in the chili. Then add in the cannellini beans and the shredded chicken. Cover the pot again and let it simmer for another 20 minutes. Turn off the heat and let the soup rest for 10 minutes. Use this time to gather your favorite chili toppings, like diced avocado, a lime wedge, a sprinkle of cheddar cheese or even gluten-free tortilla chips. Yum!

I hope this white chicken chili recipe earns a place on your wintertime menu — I know it's on mine! **By Dr. Josh Axe**

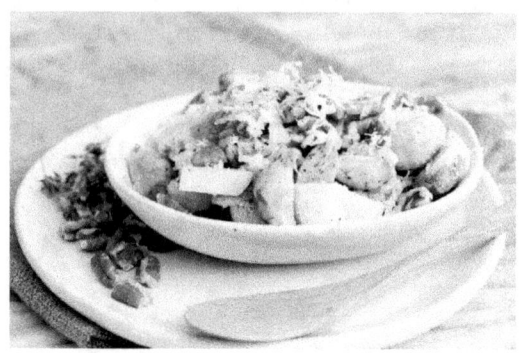

# Roasted Brussels Sprouts with Apples & Pecans

**Total Time:** 60 minutes/**Serves:** 8

INGREDIENTS:

- 2 pounds Brussels sprouts, washed, trimmed, and halved
- 2 medium shallots, minced
- sea salt and freshly ground pepper
- 1 cup white wine
- 1/4 cup ghee
- zest of 1 lemon
- 1 sweet apple, cored and diced
- 1 cup pecan pieces
- 1 teaspoon chopped fresh thyme, or 1/3 teaspoon dried
- 1/2 cup grated Zamorano cheese (optional)

DIRECTIONS:

1. Heat the oven to 350 F.
2. In a 13 x 9-inch baking dish, combine the Brussels sprouts, shallots, salt and pepper and mix together.

3. Pour the white wine into the dish and place spoonfuls of ghee on top of the sprouts, making sure all areas of the dish have ghee.

4. Bake uncovered for 30 minutes. Remove from the oven and add the lemon zest, apples, pecans, thyme and (if using) Zamorano. Stir to combine.

5. Return the dish to the oven for 15–20 minutes, or until sprouts and apple pieces are tender.

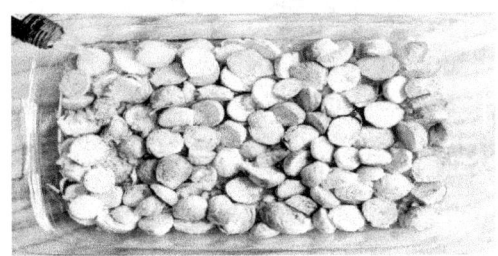

If you haven't fallen in love with Brussels sprouts yet, then this is the recipe for you. Dressed up and humble at the same time, these Roasted Brussels Sprouts with Apples & Pecans will have you wondering why you ever avoided (or maybe despised!) the tiny green cabbage.

The reason your mother or grandmother wanted you to eat **nutrition-rich Brussels sprouts** is because they are packed with antioxidants, vitamins (K, C and A are tops), minerals, fiber, omega-3s and a good amount of protein for a vegetable. Regularly eating just a one-cup serving of the cruciferous veggie can help lower your risk of cancer, strengthen your bones, protect skin and eye health, aid digestion, fight inflammation, lower glucose and cholesterol … need I go on?

This recipe adds even more vitamins and fiber with apple and the **healthy fats** of pecans and **ghee**. While Brussels sprouts, apples and pecans are at their peak in the fall and winter, they're available year-round, so try this recipe for a holiday gathering or a simple weeknight meal paired with my **Seared Grass-Fed Steak**.

Begin by heating the oven to 350 F and grabbing a 13 x 9-inch baking dish. That's the only dish you'll need for this recipe!

Add 2 pounds of trimmed and halved Brussels sprouts to the dish (we're making enough for a crowd, but you could easily half this recipe for fewer people). Throw in 2 minced shallots and some sea salt and freshly ground pepper. Mix these around so that all the veggies get some seasoning.

Next, pour in about a cup of white wine. If you want to avoid using wine, you could use chicken broth. But the wine is going to enhance the sweetness of the roasted Brussels sprouts and help them caramelize a bit.

Next top the sprouts with spoonfuls of ghee, making sure all areas of the dish have some ghee. Now pop the dish in the oven for 30 minutes. The Brussels sprouts are going to get a little browned and steamed in the wine and ghee.

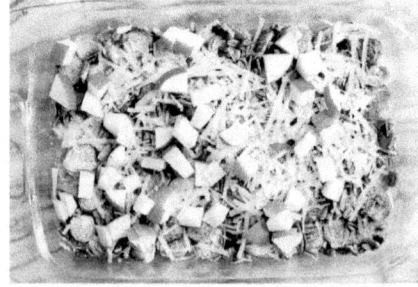

Take the dish out of the oven and add the zest of 1 lemon, 1 diced sweet apple (such as Braeburn or Fuji), 1 cup pecan pieces, and 1 teaspoon of chopped fresh thyme. You can also add 1/2 cup grated Zamorano cheese if you'd like. Zamorano is a mild, tasty cheese made from raw sheep milk, which has similar benefits as raw goat milk products.

Stir gently to combine, then its back to the oven for 15 to 20 minutes, just until the Brussels sprouts and apple pieces are tender.

Serve up these roasted Brussels sprouts while they're warm, and enjoy the sweet, nutty, tangy and buttery flavor. I love this dish with turkey or beef, but it also makes a filling veggie meal on its own and is great reheated. Their proofs that not only are Brussels sprouts incredibly good for you, they can taste incredible too. **By Dr. Josh Axe**

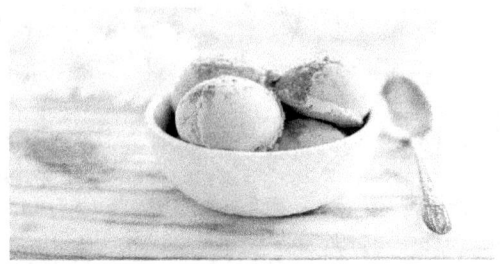

# Vegan Pumpkin Pie Ice Cream

**Total Time:** 60 minutes, plus chilling and churning time/**Serves:** 6–8

INGREDIENTS:

- 1 medium butternut squash, peeled, seeded, and diced
- pinch of salt
- 1 1/2 cans full fat coconut milk, divided
- 3/4 cup coconut sugar
- 1 teaspoon vanilla extract
- 1 sweet-tart apple, cored and sliced thick
- 1/4 teaspoon cinnamon
- 1/4 teaspoon ginger
- 1 teaspoon pumpkin pie spice
- 2 tablespoons whiskey or bourbon

DIRECTIONS:

1. Heat the oven to 425 F.
2. Line a cookie sheet with parchment paper. Spread the squash evenly on the parchment.
3. Sprinkle the squash with the salt and bake for 30 minutes. Make the coconut-caramel syrup while the squash is baking.

4. In a small pot, heat 1/2 can of coconut milk over medium-high heat. When hot, add the coconut sugar and simmer at medium heat for 6–8 minutes. Remove from the heat. Add the vanilla, stir and set aside.

5. Remove the squash from the oven. Add the apples to the pan and bake 20 minutes more

6. Remove the squash and apple from the oven and allow cooling for 10 minutes.

7. In a high-powered blender, combine the remaining can of coconut milk, coconut-caramel syrup, squash, apples, spices and whiskey/bourbon. Puree on high until thoroughly blended and thick.

8. Refrigerate in an airtight container at least 3 hours or overnight. When completely chilled, churn according to manufacturer's instructions.

9. If you're like me, there's no bad time of year to eat ice cream. Whether it's a hot summer afternoon or a lazy evening in the dead of winter, a bowl of ice cream always hits the spot.

10. But those pint prices can add up. And if you're vegan, finding dairy-free **vegan ice cream** is even more of a challenge. Unless you make my Vegan Pumpkin Pie Ice Cream, that is. Making your own chilly treat means your favorite flavor — yes, ice cream can be added to my list of favorite **pumpkin recipes** — is always in stock. You'll get added health benefits, too; try that with the store-bought brands!

11. I love the **pumpkin pie** flavor in this. It's terrific during prime pumpkin time in fall and winter, but it's delicious year-round. You might be surprised that the base of this treat is actually **butternut squash** and apples! An ice cream packed with fiber, vitamins and antioxidants? Yes, please. Add in that delicious, nutritious coconut milk and some metabolism-boosting spices, and you've got a truly guilt-free dessert.

12. Move over, Ben and Jerry. It's time to try your hand at making this Vegan Pumpkin Pie Ice Cream.

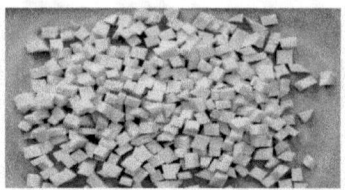

Start by cranking the oven up to 425 F and lining a cookie sheet with parchment paper for easy cleanup and no sticking. Sprinkle the diced squash with sea salt and spread onto the parchment paper.

Once the oven's ready, slide the cookie sheet in. While the squash bakes, let's go ahead and prepare our coconut-caramel syrup.

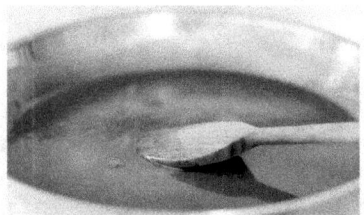

In a small pot, heat half a can of creamy **coconut milk** over medium-high heat. When it's nice and hot, add the coconut sugar. Let the coconut goodness simmer for 6–8 minutes. Remove the syrup pot from the heat and stir in the vanilla. How good does this smell? This will add a ton of flavor to our ice cream later.

Remove the baking sheet with the squash from the oven, add the sliced apples onto it and slide the sheet back into the oven. Bake 'em all up for another 20 minutes, then remove and let them cool for 5–10 minutes.

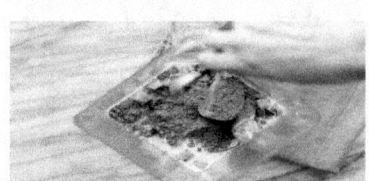

Now comes the fun part. Using a high-powered blender, add the rest of the coconut milk, the coconut syrup you made earlier, squash, apples, spices and the whiskey/bourbon. Puree all the ingredients until they're well blended and nice and thick. No one can accuse this Vegan Pumpkin Pie Ice Cream of not having any flavor.

A quick note about the whiskey/bourbon: I wouldn't skip this step unless it's absolutely necessary. Two tablespoons is a minimal-enough amount where you won't wind up with "boozy" ice cream, but it imparts a ton of taste and keeps the ice cream from freezing too hard; no one wants to eat their ice cream with an ice pick! Unflavored whiskey and bourbon also qualify as **gluten-free alcohol**.

Time for the final step: refrigerate the mix for at least three hours or overnight. When it's totally chilled, churn it all up in your ice cream maker according to the manufacturer's instructions.

No ice cream maker? No problem. Just be sure to whisk the ice cream really well before freezing, as air is an important ingredient in ice cream (weird, huh?). And no matter how you make it, let the ice cream thaw for 5–10 minutes before serving, as coconut ice creams freeze really hard — don't break a spoon!

There you have it! Super creamy, Vegan Pumpkin Pie Ice Cream. Serve with your favorite toppings and enjoy. **Recipe by Dr. Axe**

# Breast Cancer Sites

http://breastcancerconqueror.com

https://partners.emergingmed.com/options4breastcancer?utm_source=facebook&utm_medium=cpc&utm_campaign=BreastCancer&utm_term=supporter_dsktp

https://www.youtube.com/watch?v=I_djR1Hvy8k

http://www.lovelivehealth.com/7-amazing-benefits-lemon-water/?utm_source=facebookads&utm_medium=cpc&utm_campaign=fb_lemonwater_a_us

http://timesofindia.indiatimes.com/life-style/health-fitness/home-remedies/8-Indian-spices-that-prevent-cancer/articleshow/14863731.cms

http://www.realnews24.com/18-spices-scientifically-proven-to-prevent-and-treat-cancer/

http://www.care2.com/greenliving/the-healing-weeds-in-your-yard.html

If after all this you still want chemo and radiation. Go to Cancer Treatment Centers of America. They treat you holistically with diet, herbs and chemo. Each patient has their own team of doctors that treat them.

**My sincere hope is that you have found my testimony helpful and that you beat any disease by these tips and prayer! Remember Hebrews 11:6 "Without faith it is impossible to please God you must believe that God is and that He is a rewarder of those who diligently seek Him!**

**By Terry Board**

# Index

www.Breastcancer.org

http://www.breastcancer.org/symptoms/testing/types/endopredict-test

http://www.breastcancer.org/symptoms/testing/types/mammaprint

http://www.breastcancer.org/symptoms/testing/types/mammostrat

http://www.breastcancer.org/symptoms/testing/types/oncotype_dx

http://emedicine.medscape.com/article/2087535-overview

Prosigna Breast Cancer Prognostic Gene Signature Assay

http://www.breastcancer.org/symptoms/testing/types/mri

http://www.everydayhealth.com/contributing-writers-and-editors.aspx

http://www.everydayhealth.com/medical-reviewers.aspx

http://www.realnews24.com/18-spices-scientifically-proven-to-prevent-and-treat-cancer/

http://www.earthespice.com.au/blog/this-is-what-happens-to-your-body-if-you-eat-1-teaspoon-of-turmeric-every-day/

http://www.ncbi.nlm.nih.gov/books/NBK92774/

http://www.naturallivingideas.com/19-herbs-spices-that-fight-cancer/

https://draxe.com/ (This is where most of the Recipes came from)